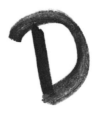

U.S. TREASURY

AMERICAN LANDMARKS

Jason Cooper

J 352.40973 COO
Cooper, Jason
U.S. Treasury

$13.95
MCFADDEN   31994011269393

The Rourke Corporation, Inc.
Vero Beach, Florida 32964

PHOTO CREDITS:
Courtesy of the Bureau of Engraving and Printing: cover, pages 7, 8, 10, 12, 15, 17, 18; Courtesy of the Department of the Treasury, Office of the Curator: title page, pages 4, 13, 21

CREATIVE SERVICES:
East Coast Studios, Merritt Island, Florida

EDITORIAL SERVICES:
Susan Albury

Library of Congress Cataloging-in-Publication Data

Cooper, Jason, 1942-
    U.S. Treasury / by Jason Cooper
      p. cm. — (American Landmarks)
    Includes bibliographical references and index.
    Summary: Discusses the United States Treasury Department, including the Bureau of Engraving and Printing, where money is printed, and the Treasury building, the oldest departmental building in Washington, D.C.
    ISBN 0-86593-550-5
    1. Money—United States—Juvenile literature. [1. United States. Dept. of the Treasury. 2. United States. Bureau of Engraving and Printing.] I. United States. Dept. of the Treasury. II. United States. Bureau of Engraving and Printing. III. Title. IV. Title: US Treasury. V. Series: Cooper, Jason, 1942- American landmarks.
HJ261.C62 1999
352.4'0973—dc21
                                  99-15316
                                      CIP

TABLE OF CONTENTS

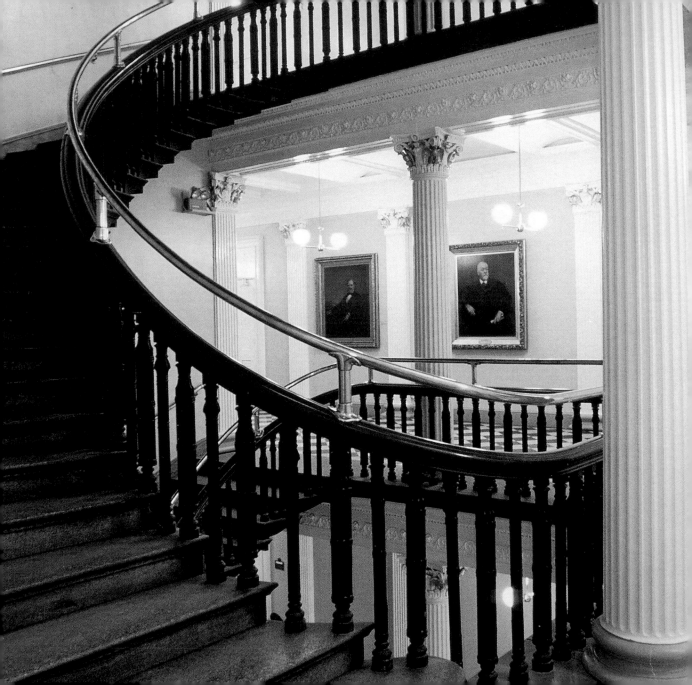

THE DEPARTMENT OF THE TREASURY

Two buildings of historic interest to Americans are part of the Department of the Treasury.

Those buildings are the Treasury Building and the Bureau of Engraving and Printing. Both are in Washington, D.C., the nation's capital.

The Treasury Building is the oldest of the **departmental** (duh pahrt MEN tul) buildings in Washington. The Bureau of Engraving and Printing is America's "money factory." Much of America's paper money, or **currency** (KUR unt see), and most of its stamps are printed here.

Winding staircases and white columns give the Treasury Building a feel of grace and beauty.

The Department of the Treasury is that part of the U.S. Government that manages the nation's money and bank accounts. Within the department are several organizations called services or bureaus. One is the Bureau of Engraving and Printing. Another is the Internal Revenue Service, or IRS.

It is the job of the Department of Treasury to print and distribute paper money. The department also **mints** (MINTS), or makes, coins. It collects income taxes from millions of Americans through the IRS. It collects the monies called **duties** (doo tees). These are monies that must sometimes be paid when foreign goods are brought into the United States.

The Bureau of Engraving and Printing prints much of America's supply of paper dollars in Washington, D.C. The bureau also produces 70 percent of America's stamps.

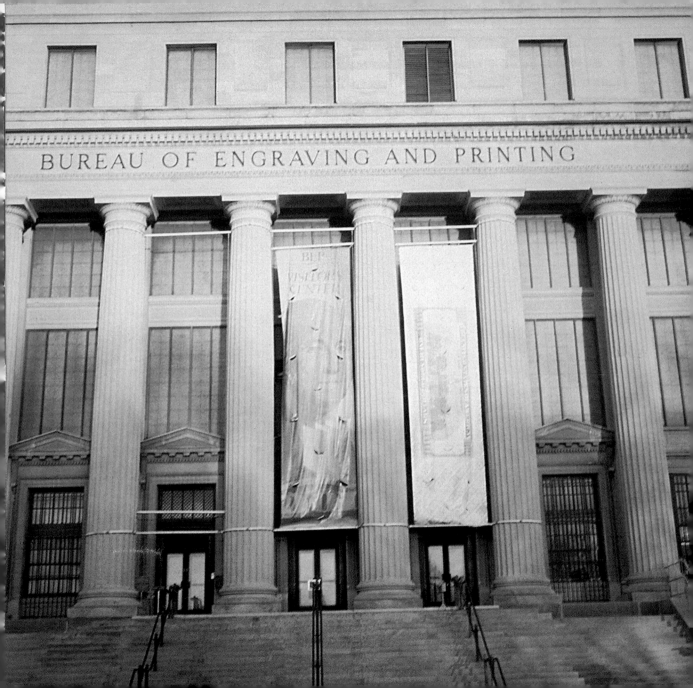

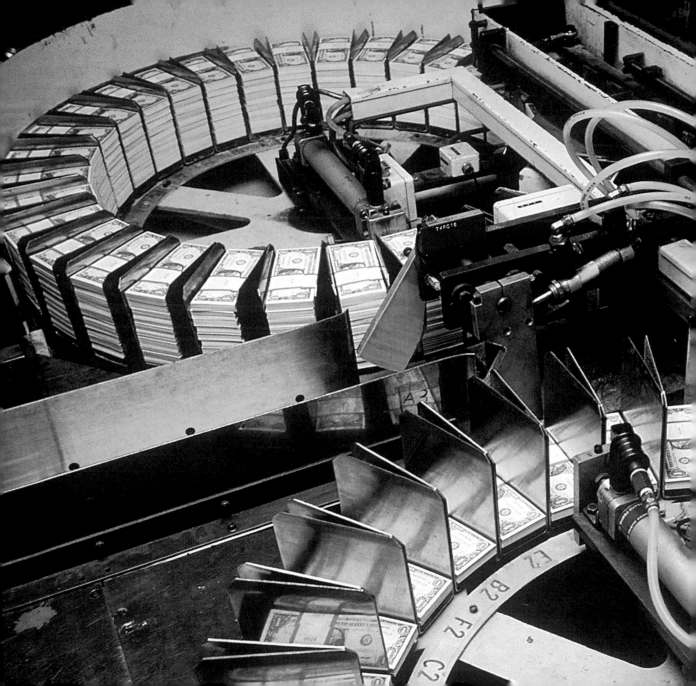

THE BUREAU OF ENGRAVING AND PRINTING

The Treasury Department job of most interest to school children is the printing of money. At the Bureau of Engraving and Printing Building, visitors can actually watch money rolling off giant printing **presses** (PRES iz).

The U.S. Government began printing paper money in 1862. The green tint to paper dollars soon earned them the nickname "greenbacks." Before the arrival of greenbacks, American currency was largely gold and silver coins.

Greenbacks are stacked at the Bureau of Engraving and Printing in Washington, D.C. The bureau is not the only site where paper dollars are printed.

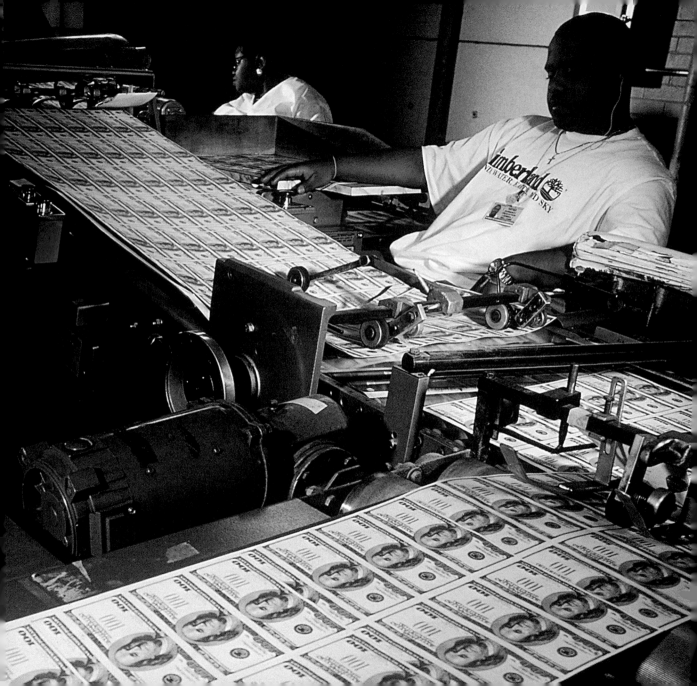

Making paper dollars in 1862 was a slow, difficult process. Six clerks in the Treasury Building basement cut the paper bills apart. Then they signed each bill and put the Treasury Department Seal on each.

The process has been greatly streamlined, but it still requires great care. Over 65 separate steps go into the process of producing paper dollars. The process begins with an artist carving into a piece of softened steel. The **engraved** (in GRAVD), or carved, steel is called a master **die** (DIE).

If you see enough of it, even money can be, well, boring. The Bureau of Engraving and Printing is America's "money factory."

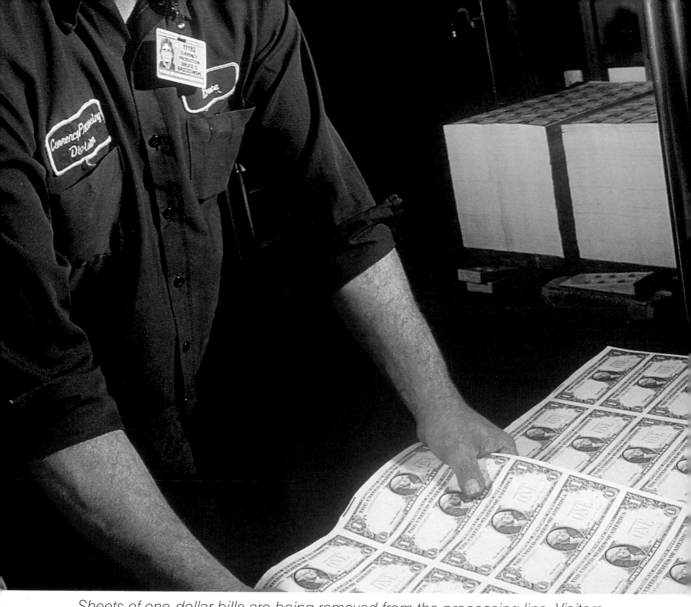

Sheets of one-dollar bills are being removed from the processing line. Visitors at the Bureau of Engraving and Printing can watch the money-making process.

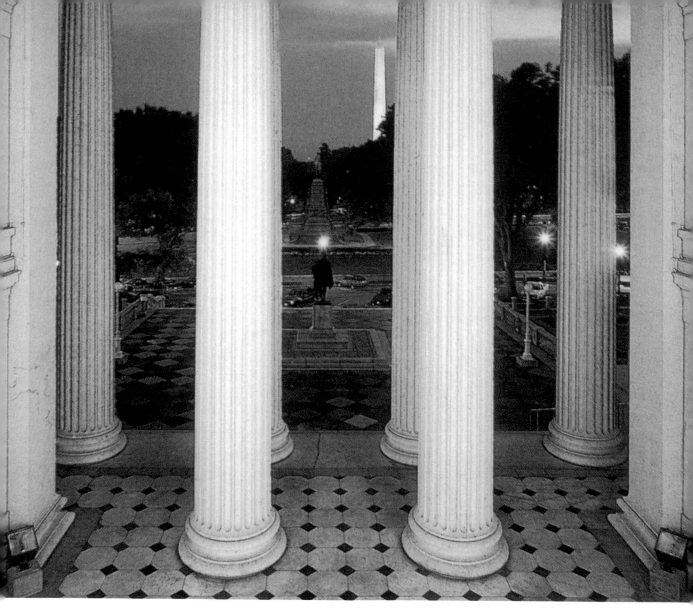

The Washington Monument can be seen through the south portico of the U.S. Treasury Building in Washington, D.C.

Images of the original die are put onto a printing plate. Money is printed from the plate. The master dies are stored. Later they can be used again.

Look at the picture of President Abraham Lincoln on a $5 bill. It was originally engraved in 1869. The engraving can still be used today.

With a type of magnifying glass called a loupe, a Bureau of Engraving and Printing designer examines a hand-engraved printing plate.

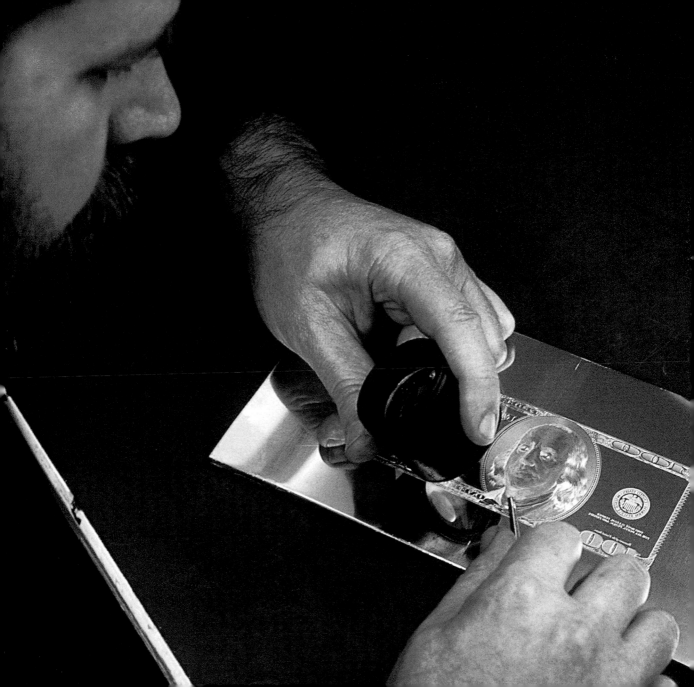

PRINTING PAPER MONEY

The Bureau of Engraving and Printing prints dollars on high-speed presses. They can print over 8,000 sheets of dollars in an hour.

The bills are first printed with ink. Then they dry for 24 to 48 hours.

Each sheet of dollars is carefully viewed by an **examiner** (ig ZAM nur). If it passes, the sheet moves along to another press. This press prints a serial number, Treasury Seal, and a federal bank seal on the bills. Cutters slice sheets into individual bills.

An examiner looks for defects in a sheet of $5 bills. Paper dollars can never show a picture of a living person.

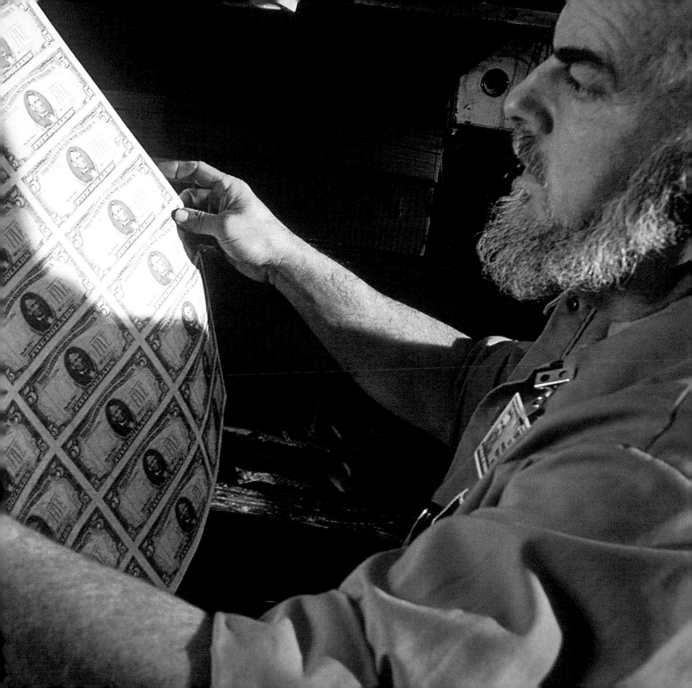

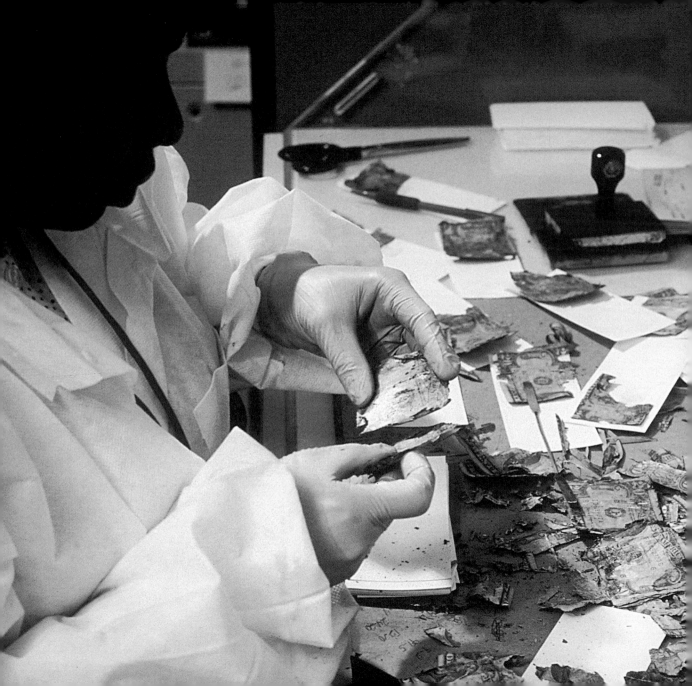

There are seven different **denominations** (duh nah mah NAY shunz), or amounts, of value on dollars: one, two, five, ten, twenty, fifty, and one hundred. Each denomination has a special design on each side. The secretary of the treasury makes the final decision about the design and the material used in the dollars.

Front designs on five of the bills show former presidents. The first secretary of the Treasury, Alexander Hamilton, appears on the face of the $10 bill.

The Mutilated Currency Division has trained people to figure out the worth of paper money that has been damaged by water, animals, chemicals, and fire.

THE TREASURY BUILDING

The present Treasury Building is a big, bold-looking building built of granite. The first Treasury Building was burned by the British in 1814. The one that replaced it was set afire and destroyed by **arsonists** (AHR sun ists) in 1833.

The present building took 33 years to complete, from 1836 to 1869. It was used as a shelter for soldiers during the Civil War (1861-1865).

The Treasury Building has 30 granite columns, each 36 feet (11 meters) tall on its eastern front.

President Andrew Johnson used this room in the Treasury Department Building as a temporary office in 1865.

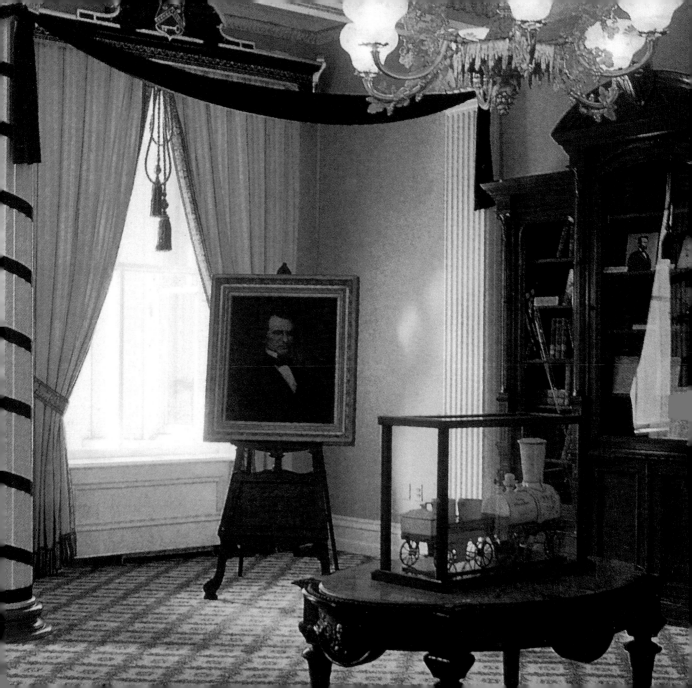

VISITING

Tours are available to both the Treasury Building and the Bureau of Engraving and Printing.

Treasury Building tours are available on Saturdays only, and reservations are needed.

The Bureau of Engraving and Printing conducts 35-minute tours daily. Visitors can watch the presses print money. They can also play money games at the visitor center and spend money at the gift shop.

GLOSSARY

arsonist (AHR sun ist) — one who purposely sets a fire to do damage

currency (KUR unt see) — money

denomination (duh nah mah NAY shun) a certain value or size

departmental (duh pahrt MEN tul) — of a certain department, such as the Department of the Treasury

die (DIE) — a tool or device that will leave its impression on something else, such as paper

duty (DOO tee) — a tax charged on goods that are brought into one country from another

engraved (in GRAVD) to have been carved with letters or figures

examiner (ig ZAM nur) — one who looks closely at an object for faults or problems

mint (MINT) — to make coins; a place where coins are made

press (PRES) a machine that prints on paper

INDEX

FURTHER READING

Find out more about money and the Department of the Treasury with these helpful books and information sites:

• Armentrout, P. *American Currency.* Rourke, 1996.
• Armentrout, P. *How Money Is Made.* Rourke, 1996.
• The Bureau of Engraving and Printing on line at www.moneyfactory.com
• The Department of the Treasury on line at www.ustreas.gov